Introduction:

Are you tired of feeling sluggish, bloated, and overweight? Do you struggle with sugar cravings or struggle to control your appetite? If so, you're not alone. Millions of people around the world struggle with their weight and overall health due to a diet high in carbohydrates, starches, and sugars.

In this book, we'll explore the benefits of a low-carb lifestyle and how it can help you lose weight, boost your energy levels, and improve your overall health. You'll learn about the science behind low-carb diets, how to plan and prepare low-carb meals and snacks, and how to stick to your low-carb lifestyle even when eating out or on a budget.

With the help of this book, you'll be able to create a sustainable low-carb lifestyle that will leave you feeling healthy, happy, and energized. So, let's dive in and explore the world of low-carb living!

Chapter 1: Introduction to the Low-Carb Lifestyle

The low-carb lifestyle has become increasingly popular in recent years, and for good reason. This diet is based on the premise that by reducing your intake of carbohydrates, starches, and sugars, you can improve your health, lose weight, and increase your energy levels.

Carbohydrates are the primary source of energy for the body, and they're found in a wide range of foods, including bread, pasta, rice, potatoes, and fruits. When we eat carbohydrates, our bodies break them down into glucose, which is then used for energy.

However, when we eat too many carbohydrates, our bodies can't use all of the glucose for energy, so it's stored as fat. This can lead to weight gain, insulin resistance, and a host of other health problems.

By following a low-carb diet, you can reduce your intake of carbohydrates and force your body to use stored fat for energy instead. This can lead to weight loss, improved blood sugar levels, and increased energy.

In the next chapter, we'll explore carbohydrates, starches, and sugars in more detail and learn which foods to avoid on a low-carb diet.

The Low-Carb Lifestyle

A Guide to a Healthy, Low-Starch, Low-Sugar Diet

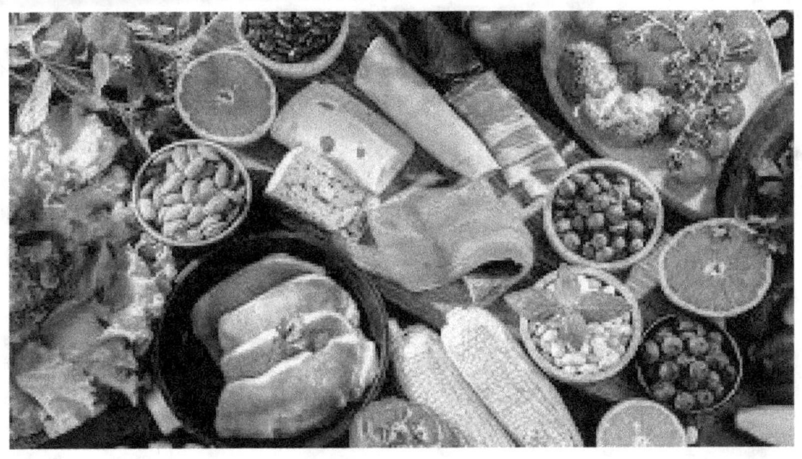

Author: Bruce Durbin

Table of Contents

Chapter 2: Understanding Carbohydrates, Starches, and Sugars

Carbohydrates are one of the three macronutrients that our bodies need for energy, along with protein and fat. There are two types of carbohydrates: simple and complex.

Simple carbohydrates, also known as sugars, are found in foods like candy, soda, and baked goods. These types of carbohydrates are quickly broken down into glucose by the body, leading to a rapid spike in blood sugar levels.

Complex carbohydrates, on the other hand, take longer to break down and provide a slower release of energy. These types of carbohydrates are found in foods like whole grains, vegetables, and beans.

Starches are a type of complex carbohydrate found in foods like potatoes, corn, and rice. Like complex carbohydrates, starches take longer to break down and provide a slower release of energy.

On a low-carb diet, it's important to avoid or limit your intake of simple carbohydrates and starches. Instead, focus on eating complex carbohydrates in moderation and getting the majority of your calories from protein and healthy fats.

Sugars are another type of simple carbohydrate that should be avoided on a low-carb diet. This includes both natural sugars found in fruit and processed sugars found in candy, soda, and other sweets.

While it's okay to eat small amounts of natural sugars in moderation, processed sugars should be avoided as much as possible. These types of sugars can lead to spikes in blood sugar levels, weight gain, and other health problems.

In the next chapter, we'll explore the science behind low-carb diets and how they can help improve your health and well-being.

Chapter 3: The Science Behind Low-Carb Diets

Low-carb diets have been around for decades, but it wasn't until recently that scientists started to study their effects on health and weight loss. Here's what the research says about low-carb diets:

1. Low-carb diets can lead to significant weight loss. Studies have shown that people who follow a low-carb diet can lose more weight than those who follow a low-fat diet. This is because low-carb diets reduce appetite and cause people to naturally eat fewer calories.
2. Low-carb diets can improve blood sugar control. By reducing carbohydrate intake, low-carb diets can help regulate blood sugar levels and improve insulin sensitivity. This is particularly important for people with type 2 diabetes.
3. Low-carb diets can lower triglycerides and increase HDL cholesterol. Triglycerides are a type of fat in the blood that can contribute to heart disease. HDL cholesterol, on the other hand, is a "good" type of cholesterol that helps protect against heart disease. Studies have shown that low-carb diets can lower triglycerides and increase HDL cholesterol levels.
4. Low-carb diets can reduce inflammation. Chronic inflammation is a risk factor for many diseases, including heart disease, cancer, and Alzheimer's disease. Some studies have suggested that low-carb diets can reduce inflammation in the body.
5. Low-carb diets can improve brain function. Some studies have shown that low-carb diets can improve cognitive function and memory in older adults.

While more research is needed to fully understand the long-term effects of low-carb diets, the evidence so far suggests that they can be a safe and effective way to improve health and manage weight.

In the next chapter, we'll discuss the benefits and drawbacks of a low-carb, low starch, low sugar diet, and how to get started on this type of eating plan.

Chapter 4: Pros and Cons of a Low-Carb, Low Starch, Low Sugar Diet

While there are many benefits to a low-carb, low starch, low sugar diet, there are also some potential drawbacks to consider. Here's a closer look at the pros and cons of this type of eating plan:

Pros:

1. Weight loss: As we mentioned earlier, a low-carb, low starch, low sugar diet can lead to significant weight loss. This is because it can reduce appetite and cause people to naturally eat fewer calories.
2. Better blood sugar control: By reducing carbohydrate intake, this type of diet can help regulate blood sugar levels and improve insulin sensitivity. This is particularly important for people with type 2 diabetes.
3. Lower triglycerides and higher HDL cholesterol: By reducing carbohydrate intake, this type of diet can lower triglycerides and increase HDL cholesterol levels. This can reduce the risk of heart disease.
4. Reduced inflammation: By reducing carbohydrate intake, this type of diet can reduce inflammation in the body. This can help reduce the risk of many chronic diseases.
5. Improved cognitive function: Some studies have shown that a low-carb, low starch, low sugar diet can improve cognitive function and memory in older adults.

Cons:

1. Restrictive: A low-carb, low starch, low sugar diet can be restrictive and difficult to follow long-term. It may also limit the variety of foods you can eat.
2. Nutrient deficiencies: If you're not careful, this type of diet can lead to nutrient deficiencies, particularly if you're not eating a variety of fruits, vegetables, and whole grains.
3. Increased risk of constipation: A low-carb, low starch, low sugar diet can be low in fiber, which can increase the risk of constipation.
4. Ketoacidosis: While rare, a very low-carb diet can cause a condition called ketoacidosis, which is a serious medical condition that can be life-threatening.

Overall, a low-carb, low starch, low sugar diet can be a safe and effective way to improve health and manage weight, but it's important to consider the potential drawbacks and speak with your healthcare provider before starting any new diet plan.

In the next chapter, we'll provide some tips and tricks for getting started on a low-carb, low starch, low sugar diet.

Chapter 5: Getting Started on a Low-Carb, Low Starch, Low Sugar Diet

If you're considering a low-carb, low starch, low sugar diet, here are some tips to help you get started:

1. Clean out your pantry and fridge: Get rid of any high-carb, high-starch, and high-sugar foods in your home, including bread, pasta, rice, sugary drinks, and snacks. Stock up on low-carb, low starch, and low sugar foods instead, such as leafy greens, low-carb vegetables, nuts, seeds, eggs, cheese, and lean meats.
2. Plan your meals: Take some time to plan out your meals for the week ahead, making sure to include plenty of low-carb, low starch, and low sugar options. This can help you stay on track and avoid impulse eating.
3. Focus on whole foods: Choose whole, unprocessed foods whenever possible, such as fresh fruits and vegetables, whole grains, and lean proteins. These foods are typically lower in carbs, starch, and sugar than processed foods.
4. Monitor your carb intake: Keep track of your carbohydrate intake by reading nutrition labels and using a food tracker app. Aim to keep your daily carb intake between 20-100 grams, depending on your individual needs and goals.
5. Stay hydrated: Drinking plenty of water is important for any healthy eating plan. Aim to drink at least 8 glasses of water per day, and avoid sugary drinks and juices.
6. Be patient: Adjusting to a low-carb, low starch, low sugar diet can take time, and you may experience some initial discomfort such as headaches, fatigue, and cravings. Be patient and stick with it, knowing that these symptoms typically improve over time.

By following these tips and staying committed to your goals, you can successfully transition to a low-carb, low starch, low sugar diet and reap the many health benefits it offers. In the next chapter, we'll provide some delicious low-carb, low starch, and low sugar meal ideas to help get you started.

Chapter 6: Low-Carb, Low Starch, Low Sugar Meal Ideas

Transitioning to a low-carb, low starch, low sugar diet doesn't mean you have to sacrifice flavor and variety in your meals. Here are some delicious meal ideas to help you get started:

Breakfast:

- Scrambled eggs with sautéed spinach and avocado
- Greek yogurt with mixed berries and nuts
- Breakfast smoothie with almond milk, spinach, berries, and protein powder

Lunch:

- Grilled chicken or fish with mixed greens and vinaigrette dressing
- Tuna or chicken salad made with Greek yogurt, celery, and almonds, served on lettuce leaves
- Vegetable soup with chicken or beef broth and low-carb vegetables like broccoli and cauliflower

Dinner:

- Grilled steak or salmon with roasted vegetables like asparagus, Brussels sprouts, or zucchini
- Spaghetti squash with meat sauce and Parmesan cheese
- Cauliflower rice stir-fry with shrimp or tofu, and low-carb vegetables like bell peppers, onions, and mushrooms

Snacks:

- Hard-boiled eggs
- Cheese and cucumber slices
- Handful of nuts or seeds

Remember, these are just a few examples of the many delicious low-carb, low starch, low sugar meal options available to you. Get creative and experiment with different ingredients and flavors to keep your meals interesting and enjoyable.

In the next chapter, we'll dive into the science behind low-carb, low starch, low sugar diets and the potential health benefits they offer.

Chapter 7: The Science Behind Low-Carb, Low Starch, Low Sugar Diets

Low-carb, low starch, low sugar diets have gained popularity in recent years as a way to promote weight loss, improve blood sugar control, and reduce the risk of chronic diseases like type 2 diabetes and heart disease. But what does the science say about these diets?

Carbohydrates, starches, and sugars are all types of carbohydrates that are broken down into glucose (sugar) in the body to provide energy. However, consuming too many carbohydrates, especially in the form of refined sugars and starches, can lead to insulin resistance and high blood sugar levels, which can increase the risk of chronic diseases.

A low-carb, low starch, low sugar diet is designed to reduce carbohydrate intake and increase consumption of healthy fats and proteins. This can lead to lower blood sugar and insulin levels, which in turn can promote weight loss and improve overall health.

Research has shown that low-carb, low starch, low sugar diets can be effective for weight loss, with some studies showing greater weight loss compared to low-fat diets. Additionally, low-carb diets have been shown to improve blood sugar control in individuals with type 2 diabetes, potentially reducing the need for medication.

Other potential benefits of low-carb, low starch, low sugar diets include improved cholesterol levels, reduced inflammation, and lower blood pressure. However, it's important to note that individual results may vary and more research is needed to fully understand the long-term effects of these diets.

It's also important to note that not all carbohydrates are created equal, and some sources of carbohydrates like fruits, vegetables, and whole grains provide important nutrients and fiber that are essential for overall health. It's important to work with a healthcare professional or registered dietitian to determine the right balance of carbohydrates, proteins, and fats for your individual needs and goals.

In the next chapter, we'll provide some tips for maintaining a low-carb, low starch, low sugar diet while dining out and traveling.

Chapter 8: Low-Carb, Low Starch, Low Sugar Eating Out and Travel Tips

Eating out and traveling can be challenging when following a low-carb, low starch, low sugar diet. However, with a little planning and some smart choices, it's possible to stick to your healthy eating habits while on the go.

Here are some tips to help you navigate eating out and traveling while following a low-carb, low starch, low sugar diet:

1. Plan ahead: Before going out to eat or traveling, research restaurant menus and look for low-carb, low starch, low sugar options. You can also pack healthy snacks like nuts, seeds, and jerky to keep you fueled on the go.
2. Choose wisely: When eating out, look for dishes that are centered around protein and healthy fats, like grilled meats or fish and salads with vinaigrette dressing. Avoid dishes that are high in refined carbohydrates like pasta, bread, and sugary sauces.
3. Request substitutions: Don't be afraid to ask for substitutions or modifications to make dishes more low-carb friendly. For example, ask for a side of vegetables instead of pasta or rice.
4. Skip the bread basket: If dining out, ask the server to skip the bread basket or bring vegetables instead.
5. Pack snacks: When traveling, pack low-carb snacks like jerky, nuts, and seeds to keep you fueled and avoid unhealthy options like fast food.
6. Stay hydrated: Make sure to drink plenty of water while traveling and dining out to stay hydrated and help control hunger.

Remember, maintaining a healthy low-carb, low starch, low sugar diet is about making smart choices and planning ahead. With a little preparation, you can enjoy healthy and delicious meals no matter where you are.

In the next chapter, we'll discuss some common misconceptions about low-carb, low starch, low sugar diets and provide some clarity on the facts.

Chapter 9: Myths and Facts about Low-Carb, Low Starch, Low Sugar Diets

There are many misconceptions surrounding low-carb, low starch, low sugar diets. Some people believe that they are unhealthy or unsustainable, while others think that they are a quick fix for weight loss. In this chapter, we'll separate fact from fiction and provide some clarity on the myths and facts surrounding low-carb, low starch, low sugar diets.

Myth: Low-carb, low starch, low sugar diets are unhealthy.

Fact: Low-carb, low starch, low sugar diets can be healthy if done correctly. A balanced low-carb diet can provide all the necessary nutrients, including protein, healthy fats, and fiber, that your body needs to function properly. However, it's important to choose nutrient-dense whole foods and avoid highly processed and sugary foods.

Myth: Low-carb, low starch, low sugar diets are not sustainable long-term.

Fact: Low-carb, low starch, low sugar diets can be sustainable long-term if done correctly. It's important to find a balance that works for you and to choose foods that you enjoy. Many people find that they feel better and have more energy when following a low-carb, low starch, low sugar diet.

Myth: Low-carb, low starch, low sugar diets are only for weight loss.

Fact: While low-carb, low starch, low sugar diets can be effective for weight loss, they are also beneficial for overall health. These diets can help improve blood sugar control, reduce inflammation, and lower the risk of chronic diseases like diabetes and heart disease.

Myth: Low-carb, low starch, low sugar diets are all about eating bacon and cheese.

Fact: While low-carb, low starch, low sugar diets can include bacon and cheese, they are not the focus of the diet. The focus is on choosing nutrient-dense whole foods like vegetables, fruits, nuts, seeds, and healthy fats like avocado and olive oil.

Myth: Low-carb, low starch, low sugar diets are difficult to follow.

Fact: While low-carb, low starch, low sugar diets may require some adjustments to your eating habits, they can be easy to follow with a little planning and preparation. There are many resources available, including meal plans, recipes, and support groups, that can help you stick to a low-carb, low starch, low sugar diet.

By separating fact from fiction, you can make informed decisions about your health and nutrition. In the next chapter, we'll discuss the importance of physical activity and exercise in maintaining a healthy low-carb, low starch, low sugar diet.

Chapter 10: The Importance of Physical Activity and Exercise in a Low-Carb, Low Starch, Low Sugar Diet

Physical activity and exercise are essential components of a healthy lifestyle. In addition to improving cardiovascular health and reducing the risk of chronic diseases, regular exercise can also enhance weight loss efforts when combined with a low-carb, low starch, low sugar diet. In this chapter, we'll explore the benefits of physical activity and exercise and provide some tips for incorporating them into your daily routine.

Benefits of Physical Activity and Exercise

Regular physical activity and exercise can provide numerous benefits, including:

1. Improved cardiovascular health: Exercise can improve heart health by reducing blood pressure, increasing HDL (good) cholesterol, and improving circulation.
2. Weight management: Exercise can help with weight loss by burning calories and building muscle mass.
3. Increased energy: Exercise can improve energy levels by boosting circulation and oxygen delivery to the muscles.
4. Reduced stress: Exercise can help reduce stress by releasing endorphins, the body's natural feel-good chemicals.
5. Improved mental health: Exercise can help reduce symptoms of depression and anxiety and improve overall mental health and well-being.

Tips for Incorporating Physical Activity and Exercise

Incorporating physical activity and exercise into your daily routine can be easy and enjoyable. Here are some tips to get started:

1. Start small: Begin with short periods of exercise and gradually increase the duration and intensity over time.
2. Find activities you enjoy: Choose activities that you enjoy, whether it's walking, biking, swimming, or dancing. This will help you stick with your exercise routine.
3. Make it a habit: Schedule regular exercise into your daily routine, just like you would any other appointment or task.
4. Mix it up: Incorporate a variety of activities and exercises to keep things interesting and prevent boredom.
5. Seek support: Join an exercise class or find a workout buddy to help keep you motivated and accountable.

Conclusion

Regular physical activity and exercise are important components of a healthy lifestyle, especially when combined with a low-carb, low starch, low sugar diet. By incorporating physical activity and exercise into your daily routine, you can improve your cardiovascular health, manage your weight, increase your energy levels, reduce stress, and improve your mental health and well-being. In the next chapter, we'll provide some tips for maintaining a healthy low-carb, low starch, low sugar diet while dining out.

Chapter 11: Tips for Dining Out on a Low-Carb, Low Starch, Low Sugar Diet

Eating out at restaurants or attending social events can be a challenge when following a low-carb, low starch, low sugar diet. However, with some planning and preparation, you can still enjoy a delicious meal while staying on track with your dietary goals. In this chapter, we'll provide some tips for dining out on a low-carb, low starch, low sugar diet.

Research the Menu

Before heading out to a restaurant, take some time to research the menu. Many restaurants now offer their menus online, so you can review the options in advance and make informed decisions about what to order. Look for dishes that are low in carbohydrates, such as salads, grilled meats, and seafood. Avoid dishes that are breaded, fried, or served with high-carbohydrate sides, such as pasta or rice.

Ask Questions

Don't be afraid to ask your server questions about the menu or how dishes are prepared. Many restaurants are happy to accommodate dietary requests, and your server may be able to make suggestions or substitutions to make a dish more low-carb. For example, you can ask for vegetables instead of potatoes as a side dish or request that your meal be prepared without any added sugars or starches.

Customize Your Order

Many restaurants allow you to customize your order to meet your dietary needs. For example, you can request that a burger be served without a bun or ask for a salad with dressing on the side. Don't be afraid to ask for modifications or substitutions to make a dish more low-carb.

Watch Your Portions

Restaurant portions are often much larger than what you would serve at home, so it's important to be mindful of how much you are eating. Consider sharing a dish with a friend or taking half of your meal home for leftovers. You can also ask for a smaller portion size or order an appetizer as your main dish.

Stick to Water or Unsweetened Beverages

Many beverages served at restaurants are high in sugar and carbohydrates, so it's important to be mindful of what you are drinking. Stick to water, unsweetened tea, or black coffee to avoid added sugars.

Conclusion

Eating out on a low-carb, low starch, low sugar diet can be a challenge, but with some planning and preparation, you can still enjoy a delicious meal while staying on track with your dietary goals. By researching the menu, asking questions, customizing your order, watching your portions, and sticking to water or unsweetened beverages, you can make informed decisions about what you eat and stay on track with your low-carb, low starch, low sugar diet. In the next chapter, we'll provide some recipes for low-carb, low starch, low sugar meals that you can prepare at home.

Chapter 12: Low-Carb, Low Starch, Low Sugar Recipes

Preparing meals at home is a great way to stay on track with your low-carb, low starch, low sugar diet. In this chapter, we'll provide some delicious and easy-to-make recipes that are perfect for those following a low-carb, low starch, low sugar diet.

1. Grilled Chicken with Vegetables

Ingredients:

- 2 chicken breasts
- 1 zucchini
- 1 yellow squash
- 1 red bell pepper
- 1 tablespoon olive oil
- Salt and pepper to taste

Instructions:

1. Preheat grill to medium-high heat.
2. Season chicken breasts with salt and pepper.
3. Cut zucchini, yellow squash, and red bell pepper into bite-sized pieces.
4. Toss vegetables with olive oil and season with salt and pepper.
5. Grill chicken for 6-8 minutes per side, or until cooked through.
6. Grill vegetables for 5-7 minutes, or until tender.
7. Serve chicken with grilled vegetables.
8. Cucumber Avocado Salad

Ingredients:

- 2 cucumbers
- 1 avocado
- 1/4 red onion, thinly sliced
- 2 tablespoons chopped fresh cilantro
- 1 tablespoon olive oil
- 1 tablespoon lime juice
- Salt and pepper to taste

Instructions:

1. Cut cucumbers into thin slices and place in a bowl.
2. Cut avocado into small chunks and add to the bowl.
3. Add red onion and cilantro to the bowl.
4. In a separate bowl, whisk together olive oil and lime juice.
5. Pour dressing over salad and toss to combine.
6. Season with salt and pepper to taste.
7. Broiled Salmon with Asparagus

Ingredients:

- 2 salmon fillets
- 1 bunch asparagus
- 1 tablespoon olive oil
- 1 clove garlic, minced
- Salt and pepper to taste

Instructions:

1. Preheat broiler to high.
2. Line a baking sheet with aluminum foil.
3. Arrange salmon fillets and asparagus on the baking sheet.
4. In a small bowl, whisk together olive oil, garlic, salt, and pepper.
5. Brush mixture over salmon and asparagus.
6. Broil for 8-10 minutes, or until salmon is cooked through and asparagus is tender.

Conclusion

These three recipes are just a few examples of the many delicious meals you can prepare on a low-carb, low starch, low sugar diet. By using fresh, whole ingredients and avoiding high-carbohydrate foods, you can create satisfying meals that are both healthy and delicious. Experiment with different recipes and ingredients to find the dishes that work best for you and your dietary goals. In the next chapter, we'll provide some additional tips and strategies for maintaining a low-carb, low starch, low sugar diet over the long term.

Chapter 13: Tips for Long-Term Success on a Low-Carb, Low Starch, Low Sugar Diet

Following a low-carb, low starch, low sugar diet can be challenging, but it's also an effective way to improve your health and manage your weight. In this chapter, we'll provide some tips and strategies to help you stick to your dietary goals over the long term.

1. Plan Ahead

One of the keys to success on a low-carb, low starch, low sugar diet is to plan your meals in advance. This can help you avoid the temptation to reach for high-carbohydrate snacks or meals when you're hungry and pressed for time. Try planning out your meals for the week on Sunday, and prepping ingredients or cooking meals in advance so that you have healthy options readily available.

2. Embrace Healthy Fats

On a low-carb, low starch, low sugar diet, healthy fats are an important source of energy and nutrients. Embrace healthy fats such as avocados, nuts and seeds, olive oil, and fatty fish like salmon. These foods can help you feel satisfied and full, while also providing important nutrients like omega-3 fatty acids.

3. Find Low-Carb Alternatives

There are many low-carb alternatives to traditional high-carbohydrate foods that can help you stick to your dietary goals. For example, cauliflower rice can be used as a substitute for traditional rice, and zucchini noodles can be used in place of pasta. Experiment with different ingredients and recipes to find low-carb alternatives that you enjoy.

4. Keep Healthy Snacks on Hand

Having healthy snacks readily available can help you avoid reaching for high-carbohydrate options when you're hungry. Some good low-carb, low sugar snack options include nuts, seeds, cheese, and hard-boiled eggs. Try keeping these snacks on hand at home and at work so that you always have a healthy option available.

5. Don't Be Too Restrictive

While it's important to limit your intake of carbohydrates, starches, and sugars on a low-carb, low starch, low sugar diet, it's also important to avoid being too restrictive. Allowing yourself the occasional treat or indulgence can help you stick to your dietary goals over the long term. Just be sure to enjoy these treats in moderation and balance them with healthy, nutrient-dense meals and snacks.

Conclusion

Following a low-carb, low starch, low sugar diet can be challenging, but with the right strategies and mindset, it can also be incredibly rewarding. By planning ahead, embracing healthy fats, finding low-carb alternatives, keeping healthy snacks on hand, and avoiding overly restrictive eating patterns, you can stay on track with your dietary goals over the long term. Remember that a healthy diet is about balance and sustainability, and focus on making small, sustainable changes that you can maintain for the rest of your life.

Chapter 14: Dealing with Social Situations on a Low-Carb, Low Starch, Low Sugar Diet

One of the challenges of following a low-carb, low starch, low sugar diet is navigating social situations that involve food. Whether it's a dinner party or a family gathering, it can be difficult to stick to your dietary goals when faced with tempting high-carbohydrate options. In this chapter, we'll provide some strategies for dealing with social situations while still sticking to your dietary goals.

1.   Be Honest with Your Friends and Family

If you're following a low-carb, low starch, low sugar diet, it's important to be honest with your friends and family about your dietary goals. Let them know that you're trying to improve your health and manage your weight, and explain that you need their support to stay on track. By communicating your goals and needs, you can help ensure that social situations are more accommodating to your dietary needs.

2.   Bring Your Own Food

One way to ensure that you have healthy, low-carb options available at social gatherings is to bring your own food. Consider preparing a dish that fits within your dietary guidelines and bringing it with you to share. This way, you can enjoy a healthy meal while still participating in social events.

3.   Focus on Protein and Vegetables

When faced with high-carbohydrate options at social gatherings, focus on filling your plate with protein and vegetables. This can help you feel full and satisfied while still sticking to your dietary goals. Look for options like grilled chicken, fish, or vegetables, and avoid high-carbohydrate sides like bread, pasta, or potatoes.

4.   Choose Your Beverages Wisely

Many social situations involve alcohol, which can be high in carbohydrates and sugar. To stick to your dietary goals, choose your beverages wisely. Consider options like wine or spirits with low-carbohydrate mixers, and avoid sugary cocktails or beer.

5.   Remember Your Goals

When faced with tempting high-carbohydrate options at social gatherings, it's important to remember why you're following a low-carb, low starch, low sugar diet.

Keep your goals in mind, and remind yourself of the progress you've made. By staying focused and committed to your goals, you can navigate social situations with confidence and success.

Conclusion

Navigating social situations while following a low-carb, low starch, low sugar diet can be challenging, but with the right strategies, it's possible to stick to your dietary goals while still enjoying social events. By being honest with your friends and family, bringing your own food, focusing on protein and vegetables, choosing your beverages wisely, and keeping your goals in mind, you can stay on track with your dietary goals and enjoy a healthy, balanced lifestyle. Remember that a healthy diet is about balance and sustainability, and focus on making small, sustainable changes that you can maintain for the rest of your life.

Chapter 15: Staying Motivated on a Low-Carb, Low Starch, Low Sugar Diet

Sticking to a low-carb, low starch, low sugar diet can be challenging, especially over the long term. In this chapter, we'll provide some tips for staying motivated and committed to your dietary goals, so you can enjoy the many health benefits of a healthy, balanced lifestyle.

1. Set Realistic Goals

When embarking on a low-carb, low starch, low sugar diet, it's important to set realistic goals that you can achieve. Don't expect to lose 20 pounds in a week, for example. Instead, set small, achievable goals that you can reach over time. Celebrate your progress and focus on the positive changes you're making, rather than the numbers on the scale.

2. Find Support

Having a support system can be incredibly helpful when trying to stick to a low-carb, low starch, low sugar diet. Look for friends or family members who are also interested in healthy eating, or consider joining a support group or online community for people following a similar diet. Sharing your experiences and successes with others can be incredibly motivating and help keep you on track.

3. Plan Ahead

One of the keys to sticking to a low-carb, low starch, low sugar diet is planning ahead. Take time each week to plan your meals and snacks, so you always have healthy, low-carb options available. Consider meal prepping, so you can have healthy meals ready to go throughout the week. By having healthy options readily available, you're less likely to be tempted by high-carbohydrate options.

4. Track Your Progress

Tracking your progress can be a powerful motivator when following a low-carb, low starch, low sugar diet. Consider keeping a food journal or using an app to track your meals and snacks, as well as your progress towards your goals. Seeing the progress you're making can help keep you motivated and committed to your dietary goals.

5. Treat Yourself

Following a healthy diet doesn't mean you can't indulge in your favorite foods from time to time. Consider allowing yourself an occasional treat, like a small piece of dark chocolate or a scoop of low-carb ice cream. By allowing yourself these treats in moderation, you're less likely to feel deprived and more likely to stick to your dietary goals over the long term.

Conclusion

Sticking to a low-carb, low starch, low sugar diet can be challenging, but with the right strategies, it's possible to achieve long-term success. By setting realistic goals, finding support, planning ahead, tracking your progress, and treating yourself in moderation, you can stay motivated and committed to your dietary goals. Remember that a healthy lifestyle is about balance and sustainability, so focus on making small, sustainable changes that you can maintain for the rest of your life. With dedication and persistence, you can achieve a healthier, happier life.